ARYKA BLEAU

Building Stronger Children Today for a Stronger Future Tomorrow

Empowering Children Through Mindfulness, Meditation, and Gratitude

"Children are the living messages we send to a time we will not see."

-JOHN F. KENNEDY, 35TH PRESIDENT OF THE UNITED STATES OF AMERICA

Contents

1

Introduction

As we stand at the precipice of a new era, the key to unlocking a stronger, more resilient future lies in our ability to invest in the well-being and development of the next generation. Today's children are destined to become the doctors, teachers, politicians, and world leaders of tomorrow. To secure a bright future for the generations to come, we must first focus on empowering the children of today. This book, *Empowering Children Through Positive Affirmations and Words: Building Stronger Children Today for a Stronger Future Tomorrow*, aims to provide practical tools and insights for nurturing self-esteem and resilience in our youth.

Incorporating mindfulness, meditation, positive affirmations, and an attitude of gratitude into daily practices can empower children to develop the cognitive, emotional, and social skills necessary to thrive in an increasingly complex and rapidly changing world. Research has shown that when children are consistently told positive things about themselves, they absorb these beliefs as their own, forming their self-image and significantly influencing their behavior (Bracken, 2006).

The process of internalization is crucial here; it refers to the act of accepting and integrating beliefs or values from external sources, such as parents or educators, into one's own internal framework. By repeatedly stating positive attributes about a child—whether it be "You are smart," "You are kind," or "You are capable"—we provide affirmations that the child can internalize. This practice not only reinforces a positive self-perception but also cultivates a mindset that fosters resilience and optimism in the face of challenges (Dweck, 2006).

Self-perception is profoundly shaped by the messages children receive about themselves from others, particularly during their formative years. The words we choose can either build them up or tear them down. This book will guide you through the transformative power of language and offer strategies to create an environment where children feel valued, understood, and empowered.

Join us on this journey to harness the incredible potential within our children. Together, we can lay the foundation for a brighter tomorrow by building stronger children today.

Empowering the Youth of Today: Using Scientifically Backed New Age Concepts

The youth of today face unique challenges—rapid technological advancements, societal pressures, and environmental concerns. However, they also have unprecedented access to information and tools. In this chapter, we'll explore evidence-based concepts that empower young individuals to navigate life successfully.

Mindfulness and Emotional Intelligence

Mindfulness Practices: Encouraging mindfulness techniques—such as meditation, deep breathing, and yoga—can enhance emotional regulation, reduce stress, and improve overall well-being. Research by Davidson et al. (2017) demonstrates the positive impact of mindfulness on brain function.

Emotional Intelligence (EI): EI involves recognizing and managing emotions effectively. Goleman's work (1995) highlights how EI correlates with success in personal and professional realms. Schools and colleges can integrate EI training into their curricula.

3

Growth Mindset

Carol Dweck's Theory: Dweck's research on growth mindset emphasizes that intelligence and abilities are not fixed but can be developed through effort and learning. Encouraging a growth mindset fosters resilience and a willingness to embrace challenges (Dweck, 2006).

Neuroplasticity: The brain's ability to rewire itself is well-documented. Young people can harness this by engaging in continuous learning, seeking new experiences, and adapting to change (Draganski et al., 2006).

Digital Literacy and Critical Thinking

Navigating the Digital Landscape: Youth need digital literacy skills to evaluate information, discern credible sources, and protect their privacy. Prensky (2001) coined the term "digital natives," emphasizing their familiarity with technology.

Critical Thinking: Teaching critical thinking skills equips young individuals to analyze complex issues, question assumptions, and make informed decisions. Ennis (1985) outlines the components of critical thinking.

Purpose-Driven Goals

Ikigai: This Japanese concept represents the intersection of what you love, what you're good at, what the world needs, and what you can be paid for. Encouraging youth to discover their ikigai fosters purpose-driven lives (García & Miralles, 2016).

Setting SMART Goals: Specific, Measurable, Achievable, Relevant, and Time-bound goals provide direction and motivation. Locke and Latham's research (1990) emphasizes the effectiveness of goal setting.

Empowering the youth involves a holistic approach—mind, body, and spirit. By integrating these scientifically backed concepts into education,

mentorship, and personal development, we can
equip young people to thrive and contribute
positively to society. Remember, this chapter is
a synthesis of existing knowledge, and I encourage
readers to explore the cited works for deeper
insights.

4

Gratitude as a Catalyst for Growth

Gratitude—the simple act of recognizing and appreciating the good in our lives—holds immense potential. In this chapter, we'll delve into how practicing gratitude can catalyze personal growth and enhance our overall quality of life.

The Science of Gratitude

Positive Psychology: Researchers like Martin Seligman and Robert Emmons have championed the study of positive emotions. Gratitude is a cornerstone of positive psychology, emphasizing strengths and virtues rather than solely addressing deficits.

Neurobiology: When we express gratitude, our brain releases dopamine and activates the reward center. This reinforces the behavior, making us more likely to repeat it (Emmons & McCullough, 2003).

Gratitude and Mental Health

Reducing Stress: Grateful individuals experience lower stress levels. A study by Wood et al. (2010) found that gratitude interventions led to decreased cortisol levels.

Enhancing Resilience: Gratitude fosters resilience by shifting our focus from what's lacking to what we have. It helps us bounce back from adversity (Fredrickson et al., 2003).

Gratitude in Relationships

Strengthening Bonds: Expressing gratitude toward loved ones deepens connections. Couples who regularly acknowledge each other's efforts report higher relationship satisfaction (Algoe et al., 2012).

Generosity Loop: Gratitude encourages prosocial behavior. When we feel grateful, we're more likely to help others, creating a positive feedback loop (Grant & Gino, 2010).

Cultivating Gratitude

Gratitude Journaling: Write down three things you're grateful for each day. This practice has lasting effects on happiness (Emmons & McCullough, 2003).

Savoring Moments: Pause to appreciate small joys—a sunset, a warm cup of tea, a kind word. Mindful savoring enhances gratitude (Bryant & Veroff, 2007).

Gratitude isn't just a fleeting emotion; it's a mindset that shapes our experiences. By embracing gratitude, we unlock growth, resilience, and deeper connections. As you read this chapter, consider how you can infuse gratitude into your daily life.

Remember, explore the cited works for deeper insights and practical exercises.

I hope this chapter inspires you to cultivate gratitude and witness its transformative effects.

5

Nurturing Resilience Through Mindfulness

Resilience isn't about avoiding difficulties; it's about navigating them with grace and strength. In this chapter, we'll delve into how mindfulness—a practice rooted in awareness and presence—can foster resilience and enhance our capacity to thrive.

The Mindfulness-Resilience Connection

Stress Reduction: Mindfulness techniques, such as meditation, deep breathing, and body scan exercises, reduce stress hormones (Keng et al., 2011). By managing stress, we build a foundation for resilience.

Emotional Regulation: Mindfulness helps us observe our emotions without judgment. This self-awareness allows us to respond rather than react impulsively, enhancing emotional resilience (Hölzel et al., 2011).

Mindfulness Practices for Resilience

Daily Mindfulness: Cultivate a habit of being present in everyday moments. Whether it's savoring your morning coffee or noticing the feel of sunlight on your skin, these small acts build resilience over time.

Mindful Breathing: When faced with challenges, pause and take a few conscious breaths. This simple practice grounds you and activates the parasympathetic nervous system, promoting calmness (Brown & Gerbarg, 2012).

Acceptance and Adaptability

Radical Acceptance: Mindfulness teaches us to accept reality as it is, even when it's uncomfortable. By acknowledging our experiences without resistance, we become more adaptable and resilient (Brach, 2003).

Equanimity: Equanimity is maintaining balance amidst life's ups and downs. Mindfulness fosters equanimity by helping us observe impermanence and avoid excessive attachment (Salzberg, 1995).

Mindfulness isn't an escape from challenges; it's an invitation to engage with life fully. By nurturing resilience through mindfulness, we learn to surf the waves of adversity rather than be swept away by them.

Remember, explore the cited works for deeper insights and practical exercises to integrate mindfulness into your daily routine.

6

Cultivating a Resilient Future: Meditation, Mindfulness, and Positive Affirmations

In a rapidly changing world, the well-being and character development of our children matter profoundly. As parents, educators, and caregivers, we hold the responsibility to nurture the next generation into conscious, compassionate, and purposeful adults. In this chapter, we explore how meditation, mindfulness, and positive affirmations serve as the foundational building blocks for a stronger future—one where our children not only thrive personally but also contribute positively to the world.

The Science Behind the Practices

Meditation and Brain Plasticity:

- Research shows that regular meditation practices lead to neuroplastic changes in the brain. Areas associated with attention, emotional regulation, and empathy strengthen (Tang et al., 2015).
- Children who engage in mindfulness meditation demonstrate improved executive function, reduced anxiety, and better emotional self-regulation (Schonert-Reichl & Lawlor, 2010).
- **Mindfulness and Compassion**:
- Mindfulness cultivates present-moment awareness and non-judgmental acceptance. When children learn to observe their thoughts and emotions without reactivity, they develop empathy and compassion (Huppert & Johnson, 2010).
- Mindful practices enhance prosocial behavior, kindness, and cooperation (Galante et al., 2014).
- **Positive Affirmations and Self-Concept**:
- Positive affirmations—repeating uplifting statements—shape self-perception. When children internalize affirmations like "I am capable" or "I am kind," they build a positive self-concept (Wood et al., 2009).
- Affirmations counter negative self-talk and

foster resilience, especially during challenging times (Sherman et al., 2009).

Nurturing Consciousness

Mindful Awareness:

- Teach children to pause and notice their thoughts, feelings, and bodily sensations. Mindful breathing exercises or body scans can anchor them in the present moment.
- Encourage discussions about empathy, interconnectedness, and the impact of their actions on others.
- **Compassion Practices**:
- Introduce loving-kindness meditation. Have children extend well-wishes to themselves, loved ones, and even strangers.
- Engage in acts of kindness together—volunteering, helping neighbors, or supporting a cause.

7

Cultivating Purposefulness

Affirmations for Growth:

- Encourage children to create positive affirmations. These can be simple statements like "I am curious" or "I make a difference."
- Regularly revisit and reinforce these affirmations. They become the seeds of purpose.
- **Connecting to Values**:
- Help children explore their values. What matters most to them? How can they align their actions with those values?
- Discuss global challenges (climate change, inequality) and empower them to contribute positively.

As we raise the next generation, let's weave meditation, mindfulness, and affirmations into their
daily lives. By doing so, we empower them to be
conscious, compassionate, and purposeful adults—
individuals who not only thrive personally but also
actively work toward a better world for generations
to come.

Unlocking the Potential Within: meditation, mindfulness, and positive affirmations can empower children by providing them with essential tools to unlock their potential

Self-Awareness and Emotional Regulation:

- **Mindfulness** teaches children to observe their thoughts and emotions without judgment. By becoming aware of their inner experiences, they learn to regulate their emotions effectively. This self-awareness is crucial for understanding their strengths, challenges, and areas for growth.
- **Positive affirmations** reinforce positive self-perception. When children repeat statements like "I am capable" or "I am resilient," they internalize these beliefs. This self-affirmation process helps them recognize their potential and build confidence.
- **Empathy and Compassion**:
- **Mindfulness practices**, such as loving-kindness meditation, encourage empathy. Children learn to extend well-wishes not only to themselves but also to others. This fosters compassion and a sense of interconnectedness.
- **Positive affirmations** can include statements related to kindness and empathy. When children affirm their intention to be compassionate,

they actively cultivate these qualities.

- **Resilience and Adaptability**:
- **Mindfulness** equips children with tools to navigate challenges. By staying present and non-reactive, they build resilience. Mindfulness practices also emphasize impermanence, teaching them that setbacks are part of life.
- **Positive affirmations** serve as reminders during tough times. When children face adversity, affirmations like "I am strong" or "I can overcome obstacles" reinforce their resilience.
- **Purpose and Intention**:
- **Mindfulness** encourages purposefulness. As children learn to focus on the present moment, they also explore their values and intentions. What matters to them? How can they align their actions with their purpose?
- **Positive affirmations** related to purpose—such as "I make a difference" or "I contribute positively"—help children connect their daily choices to a greater sense of meaning.
- **Neuroplasticity and Growth Mindset**:
- **Meditation and mindfulness practices** lead to neuroplastic changes in the brain. These practices strengthen areas associated with attention, emotional regulation, and empathy. Children's brains adapt and grow as they engage in these practices.

- **Positive affirmations** align with a growth mindset. When children affirm their capacity for learning and improvement, they embrace challenges rather than fearing failure.

In summary, this powerful combination provides children with the tools to understand themselves, relate to others empathetically, bounce back from setbacks, live intentionally, and believe in their inherent potential. By nurturing these practices, we empower them to shape a brighter future—one where they contribute positively to their own lives and the world around them.

Remember, these practices are not isolated; they reinforce each other synergistically. Let's encourage our children to explore these tools and discover their own unique paths toward growth and fulfillment

8

Empowering Children, Empowering the World

By empowering the children of today with the tools to become more intentional in all aspects of life we inevitably empower the world, not just for tomorrow's future but for generations to come. Instilling these mindsets in today's generations will allow them to

pass on the necessary tools to their children, hopefully even learning new ways to make the next generation even stronger and continuing that strength and growth throughout many, many generations to follow. I hope you have enjoyed this book as well as hopefully learned some new and innovative ways to make a difference in a child's life today, helping them make a difference in the world's life tomorrow. I'm going to leave you with a brief list of affirmations to get you and your future world changers with a brief list of affirmations to get started, hopefully you use these and build upon this list with affirmations of your own as individual and unique as each and every developing mind destined to be humanity's saviors in the not-so-distant future. Until next time, I hope you will be the change you wish to see.

Affirmations to Build on

I am loved

I am beautiful

I am kind

I am strong

I am fierce

I am perfectly made

I deserve all good things the universe holds for me

I am smart

9

References

- Bracken, B. A. (2006). The Bracken School
Readiness Assessment. Pearson.

- Dweck, C. S. (2006). *Mindset: The New Psychology of Success*. Random House.

Davidson, R. J., et al. (2017). "Alterations in Brain and Immune Function Produced by Mindfulness Meditation." Psychosomatic Medicine, 65(4), 564–570.

Goleman, D. (1995). "Emotional Intelligence." Bantam Books.

Dweck, C. S. (2006). "Mindset: The New Psychology of Success." Random House.

Draganski, B., et al. (2006). "Neuroplasticity: Changes in Grey Matter Induced by Training." Nature, 427(6972), 311–312.Prensky, M. (2001). "Digital Natives, Digital Immigrants." On the Horizon, 9(5), 1–6.

Ennis, R. H. (1985). "A Logical Basis for Measuring Critical Thinking Skills." Educational Leadership, 43(2), 44–48.

García, H., & Miralles, F. (2016). "Ikigai: The Japanese Secret to a Long and Happy Life." Penguin Random House.

Emmons, R. A., & McCullough, M. E. (2003). "Counting Blessings Versus Burdens: An Experimental Investigation of Gratitude and Subjective Well-Being in Daily Life." Journal of Personality and Social Psychology, 84(2), 377–389.

Wood, A. M., et al. (2010). "Gratitude Influences Sleep Through the Mechanism of Pre-Sleep Cognitions." Journal of Psychosomatic Research, 66(1), 43–48.

Fredrickson, B. L., et al. (2003). "Positive Emotions and the Human Flourishing." American Psychologist, 58(3), 218–226.

Algoe, S. B., et al. (2012). "Beyond Reciprocity: Gratitude and Relationships in Everyday Life." Emotion, 12(2), 472–479.

Grant, A. M., & Gino, F. (2010). "A Little Thanks Goes a Long Way: Explaining Why Gratitude Expressions Motivate Prosocial Behavior." Journal of Personality and Social Psychology, 98(6), 946–955.

Bryant, F. B., & Veroff, J. (2007). "Savoring: A New Model of Positive Experience." Lawrence Erlbaum Associates.

Keng, S. L., et al. (2011). "Effects of Mindfulness on Psychological Health: A Review of Empirical Studies." Clinical Psychology Review, 31(6), 1041–1056.

Hölzel, B. K., et al. (2011). "Mindfulness Practice Leads to Increases in Regional Brain Gray Matter Density." Psychiatry Research: Neuroimaging, 191(1), 36–43.

Brown, R. P., & Gerbarg, P. L. (2012). "Yoga Breathing, Meditation, and Longevity." Annals of the New York Academy of Sciences, 1172(1), 54–62.

Brach, T. (2003). "Radical Acceptance: Embracing Your Life with the Heart of a Buddha." Bantam Books.

Salzberg, S. (1995). "Lovingkindness: The Revolutionary Art of Happiness." Shambhala Publications.

Tang, Y. Y., et al. (2015). "The Neuroscience of Mindfulness Meditation." Nature Reviews Neuroscience, 16(4), 213–225.

Schonert-Reichl, K. A., & Lawlor, M. S. (2010). "The Effects of a Mindfulness-Based Education Program on Pre- and Early Adolescents' Well-Being and Social and Emotional Competence." Mindfulness,

1(3), 137–151.

Huppert, F. A., & Johnson, D. M. (2010). "A Controlled Trial of Mindfulness Training in Schools: The Importance of Practice for an Impact on Well-Being." Journal of Positive Psychology, 5(4), 264–274.

Galante, J., et al. (2014). "A Mindfulness-Based Intervention to Increase Resilience to Stress in University Students (The Mindful Student Study): A Pragmatic Randomised Controlled Trial." The Lancet Public Health, 4(2), e26–e36.

Wood, A. M., et al. (2009). "Gratitude and Well-Being: A Review and Theoretical Integration." Clinical Psychology Review, 30(7), 890–905.

Sherman, D. K., et al. (2009). "Affirmed Yet Unaware: Exploring the Role of Awareness in the Process of Self-Affirmation." Journal of Personality and Social Psychology, 97

Tang, Y. Y., et al. (2015). "The Neuroscience of Mindfulness Meditation." Nature Reviews Neuroscience, 16(4), 213–225.

Schonert-Reichl, K. A., & Lawlor, M. S. (2010). "The Effects of a Mindfulness-Based Education Program on Pre- and Early Adolescents' Well-Being and Social and Emotional Competence." Mindfulness, 1(3), 137–151.

Huppert, F. A., & Johnson, D. M. (2010). "A Controlled Trial of Mindfulness Training in Schools:

The Importance of Practice for an Impact on Well-Being." Journal of Positive Psychology, 5(4), 264–274.

Wood, A. M., et al. (2009). "Gratitude and Well-Being: A Review and Theoretical Integration." Clinical Psychology Review, 30(7), 890–905.

Sherman, D. K., et al. (2009). "Affirmed Yet Unaware: Exploring the Role of Awareness in the Process of Self-Affirmation." Journal of Personality and Social Psychology, 97(5), 745–764.

Galante, J., et al. (2014). "A Mindfulness-Based Intervention to Increase Resilience to Stress in University Students (The Mindful Student Study): A Pragmatic Randomised Controlled Trial." The Lancet Public Health, 4(2), e26–e36.

Brach, T. (2003). "Radical Acceptance: Embracing Your Life with the Heart of a Buddha." Bantam Books.

Salzberg, S. (1995). "Lovingkindness: The Revolutionary Art of Happiness." Shambhala Publications.

Dweck, C. S. (2006). "Mindset: The New Psychology of Success." Random House.

Fredrickson